Essent

Complete Guide for Aromatherapy

Learn How To Use Essential Oils for A Healthy Life

By: Denise Williams

9781632874573

PUBLISHERS NOTES

Disclaimer – Speedy Publishing, LLC

This publication is intended to provide helpful and informative material. It is not intended to diagnose, treat, cure, or prevent any health problem or condition, nor is intended to replace the advice of a physician. No action should be taken solely on the contents of this book. Always consult your physician or qualified health-care professional on any matters regarding your health and before adopting any suggestions in this book or drawing inferences from it.

The author and publisher specifically disclaim all responsibility for any liability, loss or risk, personal or otherwise, which is incurred as a consequence, directly or indirectly, from the use or application of any contents of this book.

Any and all product names referenced within this book are the trademarks of their respective owners. None of these owners have sponsored, authorized, endorsed, or approved this book.

Always read all information provided by the manufacturers' product labels before using their products. The author and publisher are not responsible for claims made by manufacturers.

This book was originally printed before 2014. This is an adapted reprint by Speedy Publishing, LLC with newly updated content designed to help readers with much more accurate and timely information and data.

Speedy Publishing, LLC

40 E Main Street,

Newark

Delaware

19711

Contact Us: 1-888-248-4521

Website: http://www.speedypublishing.com

REPRINTED Paperback Edition: ISBN: 9781632874573

Manufactured in the United States of America

DEDICATION

This book is dedicated to my mentor and best friend Mindy. She taught me how to use aromatherapy oils and I thank her for that.

In eth long run natural choices really do work out better when it comes to health and wellness.

TABLE OF CONTENTS

INTRODUCTION

Aromatherapy has been considered down through the century as a remedy that soothes the body and mind. The remedies are said to relieve symptoms coming from a variety of diseases. In addition, the remedies are claimed to relieve stress, anxiety, nervous tension, and related symptoms. Many people have used aromatherapy, including the French natives, Egyptians, Germans, Brazilians, Europeans, Indians, Canadians, Americans, people in the Mediterranean lands, and so on.

The oils include the scented and essential oils. Online you can find a variety of the oils, including Basil, Cedar wood, celery seed, carrot seed, African Bluegrass oils, bergamot, clove bud and leaf oils, and so on. The oils each have its purpose for healing the body and mind. Before using the oils, be sure to read all available instructions before using.

CHAPTER 1- AROMATHERAPY-A BRIEF HISTORY

Aromatherapy came from France, which a Frenchman burnt his arm, dipped it in lavender oil, and concluded from the results that essential oils and scented oils are healers. The result delivered ceased the burning, as well there were no apparent scars on his arm. Essential oils and scented oils are aromatherapy oils, which came from living plants. Exceptions include the oils that came from swallowtail butterflies.

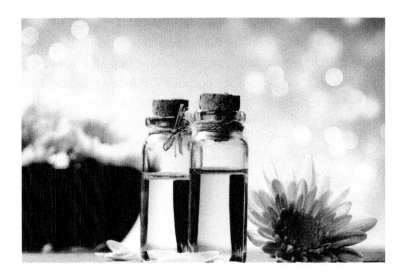

The intentions of the oils are to heal the body and mind by relaxing the soul of stress. Few types of oils are intended to produce a romantic mood. However, according to reports the best alternative for using aromatherapy comes from massaging the oils into the flesh.

I've talked with a masseuse who claims that many of her clients complained, since the oils made them feel drowsy, or put them to sleep. Consequently, the oils must work to relax the body and mind; otherwise the person would not feel drowsy or sleep when the oils are burning. The masseuse also mentioned that the green oils were prone to relax the body and mind, more so than other scents. Now, whether this is true or not would depend on the person and his or her level of stress.

As for aromatherapy creating romantic mood well the fact is down through the years candle lit dinners, candle lit areas, etc have created a romantic mood for many. So we can assume that aromatherapy can also create a romantic mood. The romantic oils include Jasmine. Still, a selection of aromatherapy oils can work as a romantic sparker.

Understand that aromatherapy romantic oils are essential oils. The oils work to create synchronization with the spirit, mind, and body. The oils are said to elevate moods through feeling by producing relaxation affects. The affects are said to enhance well-being, confidence, and openness. According to studies, few people using essential oils experienced a hormonal affect, which increased desire of sexuality.

The oils available to promote romance are the Patchouli oils, YLANG YLANG oils, Sandalwood, Jasmine, etc. The oils are said to deliver a strong arousing feeling. The oils work by sending odors that stimulate the moods and mind, which in turn produces an arousing sensation, as well as an awakening yearning. Aromatherapy oils with aphrodisiac ingredients are also romantic arousers. YLANG, Lemon oils, Patchouli, Rosewood, Eucalyptus, Geranium, and Rosemary are a few of aromatherapy oils, which contain aphrodisiac. Aphrodisiac Sensual oils are oil that produces a romantic mood.

How Do I Choose Oils for Massaging?

Essential Oils Bible

Distilled oils, which are made from low temperatures and pressure, as well as 100% natural graded A, oils is ideal for romantic massages. According to reviews however, you should dilute the oils in the carrier oil. Carrier oils is said to affect the skin, which produces relaxation. Additional oils include the romance oils. The oils contain cedar wood, clove buds, cinnamon leaf, clary sage, orange, and chamomile.

Yohimbe oils which include the Combinations work by increasing erectile capabilities, libido, and sex drives.

How Do I Choose the Types of Oils for Different Occasions?

You should learn more about the scents and essential oils to make your choice. Lavender oils work to balance, elucidate, soothe, and regularize the body and mind. Eucalyptus oils work to purify, cool, balance, and revitalize the body and mind. Peppermint oils invigorate, refresh, cool, and promote energy whereas Rosemary revitalizes, warms, and clarifies the body and mind. Sweet Orange oils uplift your body and mind, as well as produce a cheerful and stimulating feeling. Geranium lifts, balance, stabilizes and relaxes the body and mind. Bergamot oils lift your moods, normalize your mind, and build your confidence.

CHAPTER 2- WHAT IS AROMATHERAPY?

Aromatherapy is an alternative medicinal remedy, which is related to CAM. (Complementary & Alternative Medicine) Aromatherapy is made up of liquid plants, or materials. Aromatherapy can be found in the essential and scented oils area. The aromatic scented oils are another area was you will find aromatherapy. The mixture of plants is said to have an effect on health and moods.

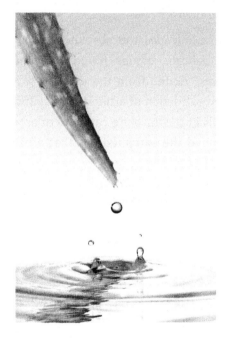

Aromatherapy has been in existence for some time. The oils were quickly put on the market after a French man discovered that the oils could heal burns without scarring the flesh. He had suffered a dramatic burn while working in his laboratory, which immediately he dipped his arm in lavender oils. He got good results, which lead to aromatherapy and the notion that it can heal the body and mind.

Aromatherapy comprises a set of branches. The branches include perfumes, self treatments, home therapy, cosmetic usage, clinical therapy, pharmacology, pharmacotherapy, Aromacology, etc. Aromacology is the process of healing the psyche by using odors and scents that affect the mind.

Aromatherapy includes essential oils, which are fragrances that were extracted from living plants. The extracting process produced aromatherapy through distillations, which included eucalyptus oils. Grapefruit oils were also produced through distillations of plants.

Aromatherapy also includes the absolute fragrances which were extracted from delicate tissues found in plants, and flowers. Aromatherapy was created from these sources through a solvent process or else an extraction of artificial fluids. Rose fluids made up Rose Essential Oils in the absolute category of aromatherapy. Rose Fragrances described the extracted oils that arose from concrete, scented butter, ethanol, etc.

Aromatherapy includes the PHYTONCIDES. The organic volatile compounds came from the roots of plants, which were utilized to annihilate microorganisms, also known as microbes. The oils are based from terpene, or sulfuric plant compounds. Terpene is the larger class of diverse hydrocarbons. The carbons are produced in living plants, which includes the prime plant life, such as the conifer.

Conifer is a cone bearing tree. In addition, carbons may also arrive from insects. The prime insects may include the swallowtail butterfly. Carbon is also a chief constituent deriving from turpentine, and resin. Turpentine is the prime source, where terpene got its name. Terpene then is a prime ingredient found in essential oils. You can use essential oils to add flavor to foodstuff, perfumes, aromatherapy, etc.

In addition, hydrosol is a variant of aromatherapy. Hydrosol is a watery incidental product, which was distilled in Rose water. This is the scented oils you can find in aromatherapy lanes. Hydrosol limits itself to CAMOMILES and Roses. The purpose of limitation is that hydrosol is a colloidal solvent, which particles are often suspended in water, and sometimes the fragrance is unfriendly.

Aromatherapy also includes infusions. Infusion is another watery extract deriving from living plants. Infusion often comes from CHAMOMILE. Aromatherapy includes Carrier oil. The oil is extracted from TRIACYLGLYCERIDE, and is diluted and produced as essential oils. Sweet Almond Oils is one of aromatherapy's oils, which came from carrier oils. The oil is utilized to treat the skin.

How Do I Know If Aromatherapy Will Work For Me?

You don't. Most times people have to use a large volume of scents and oils to produce good results, according to reviews. However, theorists have made many claims related to aromatherapy. In addition, many have tried the scented oils and essential oils, which the results led to practitioners using the oils as an herbal solution, naturopath, medicinal remedy for infections, healing aids, etc. According to reports, the oils work best when massaged into the skin, since it will set in motion the limbic system, as well as the emotional section. In addition, aromatherapy was known to set in motion the thermal receptors. There is nothing like relaxing with the smells of aromatherapy.

CHAPTER 3- EXTRACT TO HEAL WITH AROMATHERAPY

Aromatherapy works to heal the mind and body. The natural herbs, oils, fragrances, etc aid in healing a wide array of diseases. At most aromatherapy reduces irritating symptoms, as well as emotional negativity's. Aromatherapy is used to heal the mind by relieving stress.

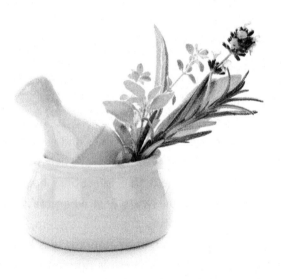

Down through the century's aromatherapy has been used by a wide selection of professionals and individuals alike. India natives, Egyptians, Germans, Frenchmen, Europeans, Brazilians, etc, have all used and still use aromatherapy oils. After ongoing studies, research, etc, the oils has proven to assist in promoting health. In fact, medical doctors use aromatherapy in medical treatment. On the market is a variety of aromatherapy scented and essential oils.

The oils include asafetida, Cajuput, Celery Seed, Jasmine, Black Currant Seed, Carrot Seed, Bergamot, Basil, and so on. Absinthe, Ajowan, African Bluegrass, Anise Star, Anethi, Australian Balm Mint Bush, Arborvitae Wild are a variety of other oils available on the market.

Australian Balm Latin name is Prostandthera Melissifolia. The flowery plant was extracted through steam process. The oils origin is Australia, which its flowers is shaped similar to a purple bell. The oils are pale yellow once extracted, and works as an anti-bacterial agent. The oils work as anti-fungal agents as well. Australian Balm will help reduce colic, headaches, and colds. The medium scented oil blends with peppermint, lavender, lemongrass, spearmint, and citronella. The oils are non-toxic and are used as a cooking ingredient as well.

Ajowan is an essential oil, which its Latin name is Trachyspermum Copticum. The herbs were extracted through a steam distillation process. The origin of ajowan starts in India. Ajowan produces pale, yellowish brown oils. The oils are essential for stimulating, and are used as anti-spasmodic agents. In addition, ajowan has microbial agents, and properties that help to fight colic symptoms. The strong scent blends with sage, thyme, and parsley.

Ajowan is sometimes called Bishop Weed. The oils originated in India, yet they are widely used in Egypt, Iran, Afghanistan, and Pakistan. You must dilute the oils before applying to the skin, otherwise it could cause irritation. If you're pregnant it is recommended that you do not use the oils.

Anise Star in Latin is called Illicium Verum. The oils are extracted through steam distillation process, and come from plant seeds. In addition, Anise Star originates in China, yet it has a well-known usage in various lands. Anise is a plant that grows licorice flavored seeds. The Mediterranean plants are used in medicines, and to flavor drink and foods. The Latin name is Pimpinella Anisum. The oils are clear, or light yellow. Moreover, the oils are used to treat colic, rheumatism, and are used in cough syrups, as well as pastille. The light scented oils blend with orange, lavender, pine, clove, cinnamon, and rosewood. The oil is used in various lands as well as a breath freshener and aid to clear up the digestive system.

Arborvitae Wild is an essential oil, which its botanic name is Thuja OCCIDENTALIS. The extraction of the needle and twigs from plants occurred through a steam distillation process. The origin of these plants is Canada. Arborvitae Wild is a confer tree, which is akin to the cypress family. The flat leaves fit closely, which the leaves resemble scales.

The oils are pale yellow, which the oil is used as an anti-rheumatic agent, anti-infection solution, anti-allergenic aid, etc. The oil is also used as an insect repellent. In addition, you can use this oil as an anti-inflammatory agent, to treat poison ivy, as an anti-microbial agent, etc. The strong scented oils blend with cinnamon Bark, birch sweet, eucalyptus, cedar wood, cajuput, and cassia oils. Arborvitae Wild is considered the oils of from the trees of life. The oils were used to ward off lightning. Arborvitae Wild oils are to be used as instructed. We can now learn how to use aromatherapy.

CHAPTER 4- HOW IS AROMATHERAPY USED?

While aromatherapy is made up of natural ingredients, it is smart to use the remedies as recommended. Some of the essential oils can cause nausea, vomiting, skin irritation, etc. Since we have a variety of articles available discussing aromatherapy oils and how they work, I thought we could switch up and learn how to use aromatherapy. Absinthe is one of the essential oils available.

How to use Absinthe:

You should use absinthe oils as instructed. The oils include cautions, which recommend that you do not use absinthe with aromatherapy treatments. The oils have agents that work against aromatherapy, such as neurotoxin, thujone, etc.

Absinthe is dark green oil, which is commonly used to treat anorexia. As well, the oil is used to boost the digestive system, while promoting menstruation. In addition, the oil is used to reduce fever, as well as remove worms. The strong scents do not blend with other oils at this time. The prime use of absinthe was to eliminate tapeworms. A last word of caution on absinthe is that people down through the years found that it could be used as a drug for getting high.

African Bluegrass is an essential oil. The oils can cause irritation to the skin. You should also avoid using the oils around the eyes. African Bluegrass is used as an astringent, anti-fungal agent, antiviral agent, and is prepared and used to sooth the feet. The medium scent oils or strong scent blend with floral and citrus notes.

Angelica Root is another of the essential oils, which pregnant women should avoid. The oils are non-toxic; however it is recommended that you avoid using the oils in sunlight. The oil is commonly used in treating gouty, arthritis, joint discomfort, congested skin, nervous tension, migraines, bronchitis, fatigue, water retention, coughing, stress disorders, and so on. The strong scents blend with sandalwood, Cedarwood, Olibanum, and Guaiacwood.

Armoise Mugwort oils should be diluted before usage, since it is toxic oil. The oils include neurotoxin and arbort-ifacient agents. Pregnant women should avoid using this oil. The oil is used as an antispasmodic, and to treat colic based symptoms. IN addition, the oil is used to discharge worms, reduce stomach acids, and so on. The strong scented oil works with oak moss, patchouli, pine, lavender, Rosemary, Clary Sage, sage, Cedarwood, and so on. You can find this oil listed in Felon Herb lines as well. St. Johns line may also have this oil listed.

Aromatherapy has a long line of essential and scented oils. Yet, each, oil has its instructions, which you should follow to avoid harm. The oils are intended to relieve the mind and body, which some oils are taking orally, while others are not.

Bay essential oils is commonly used as an antiseptic, analgesic, antibiotic, astringent, anti-neuralgic, insecticide, febrifuge, sedative, and so on. The oils are claimed to treat colds, rheumatism, flu, muscle pain, skin infections, dental infections, diarrhea, circulation irregularities, neuralgia, and so on. The strong scented oil works with juniper, Cedarwood, ginger, Ylang oils, geranium, coriander, lemon oils, eucalyptus, lavender, Rosemary, rose, thyme, and orange flavored oils. Bay essential oils is highly concentrated with Eugenol, which can irritate the flesh, mucus membrane, and so on. It is recommended that the oils are used as recommended and that pregnant women avoid using the oils.

A variety of other aromatherapy oils are available, including cardamom, bergamot, caraway, bergamot-Bergaptene free oils, Cananga, Betal Leaf, birch in both tar and sweet oils, cajuput, Cade, black currant seed oils, Calamus root, Buchu, blood orange, Cabreuva, Camphor, Cypress Australian Blue, Basil, and so on. Aromatherapy includes the essential and scented oils.

Curing with Aromatherapy

Imagine the sweet smells of aroma coffee perking in the coffeemaker. Each morning when you arise you smell those sweet aromas that perk your nostril. Well know you can add to that smell by using aromatherapies botanical COFFEA ARABICA, or coffee essential oils. The aromas were extracted from coffee beans, or plants. The flavors derived from Brazil. The coffee oils in aromatherapy provide you a smell similar to what you experience from brewed coffee. You smell the aroma and start to feel invigorating and warm.

Coffee aromas are described as the earlier cultivations where as the class of coffee trees where grown often. The species included CANEPHORA and ARABICA, which are fine coffees. Coffee aromatherapy is dark oils, which the coffee oils when burned will deodorize the environment. Coffee is found to be a great antioxidant. Coffee oils work to help those smelling the aromas reduce depressive symptoms. Coffee is also found to soothe respiratory complications, fevers, bee or bug stings, nausea, etc.

Coffee oils is unlike other aromatherapy aromas in that the coffee oils work best alone. Typically you can find coffee aromas in medium or thick formulas. The strength of the aromas is typically medium or strong scents.

The history of coffee oils spaces out. While minimal information is available, the Islamic Monks once utilized coffee oils, especially when one monk found it hard to stay alert while praying. He spotted a man in a field, which appeared gleeful and asked the man what was his recommendation. The man recommended the aromatic smell of coffee, coffee beans, or oils. The man bent on finding alertness took comfort in coffee aromas, which sparked the entire congregation. Africans, Chinese, Brazilians, Latino, Dutch, etc, including America all found it easier to stay awake while consuming or smelling coffee beans. Coffee is an Abyssinian name, which is called CAFFA.

Cyproil is another of the dark aromas. The botanical CYPERUS SCARIOSUS oil came from flower parts, which were extracted via steam. The oils come from Brazil, just as the coffee beans. Cyproil oils are grassy oil, which aromatic floral scents circle the air. The oils are light brown, or dark amber colored. Cyproil is commonly utilized as a perfume, which includes soaps, incense sticks, etc. The oils work as well as a repellant to ward off insects, as well as a healing medicine. Cyproil oils include the spicy oils, wood, earth, etc. The oils will blend with other aromatic oils, such as Clary Sage, Bergamot, Patchouli, and Labdanum. This particular oil was also used in the India lands, which the purpose was to reduce digestion complications.

Cade oils fall along the essential oil line. The oils are botanical Juniperus Oxycedrus, which the oil is made from woods and distilled via steam. The aromatic derived from France, which it too is darker colored oil. Cade oils come from evergreen shrubs. Cade oils are extracted from the heartwoods and braches where needled shrubs grow black berries.

Cade oils are commonly used as a liniment or ointment. The oils treat severe skin conditions, eczema, PRURIGO, parasitic, psoriasis, ringworms, etc. In addition, the oils are used as disinfectants, antiseptics, antimicrobial, anti-pruritus, vermifuge, analgesics, parasiticides, etc. You can find medium aromas which blend with Clove Bud, Thyme, Cedar Wood, Labdanum, Rosemary, and Origanum. The odors produced by Cade include tar aromas, smoke, dry, etc, the oils are non-toxic. The oils were commonly used in areas of France; however Africa and Europe now use the oils.

CHAPTER 5- ESSENTIAL OILS & AROMATHERAPY

Aromatherapy includes the scented oils. As well aromatherapy includes the essential oils. The oils work by melting away your stress while the aroma fragrances relax the body, as well as the mind. Aromatherapy is essentials and natural oils. The therapeutic oils allow you to utilize its fragrances in a variety of ways. Aromatherapy oils soothe your body, whilst spoiling the soft tissues of the body and relaxing the mind.

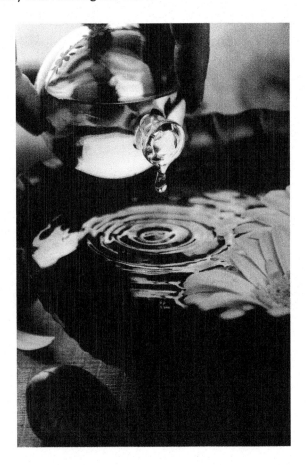

Denise Williams
How to Find Aromatherapy Scented and Essential Oils?

Online you can find a wide assortment of your favorite oils. The oils and scents wash away the days stress. Aromatherapy is the choice which helps you to relax. In addition, you can use aromatherapy oils to set a romantic mood. The oils create a loving feeling, which each of your will experience. In summary, aromatherapy will provide you a relaxing moment in a romantic setting. Oils are also handy for decorating warmers, or mists, since aromatherapy oils fill your environment with natural and fresh scents.

Scented and Essential Oils create a peaceful environment. Aromatherapy scented oils also works to enhance moods in your home environment. Scented oils naturally generate sensual and loving moods, as well as a feeling of relaxation. In fact, many masseuses' will employ aromatherapy combined with reflexology, manipulation massages, and so on. The oils help to relax the body and mind, while setting the mood.

Oils for Romantic Evenings

IF you want to set the mood for both you and your partner, thus Jasmine is the ultimate aromatherapy. Jasmine includes the Queen oils, which is aromatherapy's essential oils. The scented aromas will set the mood, by producing a luxurious scent. The scent works to create a loving bond between you and your mate. The uninhibited aromatherapy oil is irresistible and will put you and your partner both in the mood.

Aromatherapy oils produce scents which surround your environment. The scented oils will appeal to moods, memory, appetite, body, mind, etc. You've almost certainly took notice of the advertisements, which informed you of exotic, aromatherapy, scented, or essential oils. However, aromatherapy, oils are natural oils, which differ from other types of oils. Aromatherapy comes in a variety of scents, including "Jasmine, Cedar, Lilac, Tuberose, and Myrrh. You have options however, since can purchase a variety of natural scents, such as the enthralling natural forest oils and floral scents.

Those feeling cheerful may benefit from the warmth of fig oils. The oils will keep you in your cheerful mood. The warmth of fig oils includes the orange and cinnamon scents.

The aromatherapy scents set the natural feeling or moods. You merely smell the oils. In addition, the oils will supply new age solutions, since you can use aromatherapy as air fresheners.

Why Choose Aromatherapy over Common Oils?

Common oils incorporate chemicals, which will affect the body. You will perhaps experience sinus problems, or related problems using common oils. In addition, aromatherapy oils set the mood in a natural environment. Aromatherapy oils produce sweet smells in the air. Still, the scents will not affect your sinuses or skin. Moreover, you will not need to invest in products sold at local stores, which the unnatural fresheners will only freshening your home for a short time.

Online you can find a wide assortment of aromatherapy oils. The oils again include the essential oils, and scented oils. Make sure you understand the difference, since each aromatherapy scented or essential oils produce a different effect. For instance, few oils are designed to spark romance, while other oils are designed to lift your moods.

Questions of the Day

You've probably read scores of articles related to scent and essential oils, which arrive from aromatherapy. Probably what you haven't read is articles informing you how the vendors decide on which oils to purchase for resell. Since, you may have not read such articles will consider vendors. Why...because how vendors decide can also help you decide which aromatherapy oils are right for you.

How do vendors decide which scented and essential oils are best for marketing?

Vendors typically consider flavor, medium utilized for sell, targeted selections sold in society, purpose intended, cost, etc.

Base idea:

Scented and essential oils, such as the aromatherapy oils work to melt away daily stress. The fragrances work to relax the body and mind, which provides a healing aid. Aromatherapy essential oils and scented oils are organic oils that derived from living plants. The therapeutic oils make it easy for you to take advantage of its scents in a variety of ways. Aromatherapy scented and essential oils soothe the body and mind, at the same time the oils pamper the skin. Vendors and purchasers choose their favorite oils and designer fragrances based on the volume sold. The aromatherapy oils assist those with overwhelming stress, by relaxing the mind and body. In addition, vendors look for the oils that put you in a romantic mood. Vendors and purchasers alike know what people like.

In addition, vendors and purchasers tend to search for decorative home warmers or misted oils that fill the environment with fresh and natural fragrances. People tend to enjoy the great outdoors.

How long have vendors sold aromatherapy oils?

Scented and essential oils or fragrance have been utilized for 100 years in one fashion or the other. The oils were utilized to keep a pleasing odor in our homes and/or our work environment. In addition, purchasers use the oils to freshen their vehicle. At one time the oils were available in selective flavors. Nowadays however vendors and purchasers alike can choose from hundreds of flavors varying from apple to orange. African rain and Ylang-Ylang oils are also available.

The Chinese started using the oils whilst promoting the oils as energy enhancers. Indians enjoyed aromatherapy oils, since the oils were praying tools that aiding in what they believed their god would hear from special oils dipped in wax sticks, which they called agarbatti. Thus, the Indians believed that the oils would create a spiritual milieu. The special oil flavored candles are available today which are used for aromatherapy, similar to what the Indians used.

How do vendors and purchasers test aromatherapy oils?

Vendors and purchasers alike tend to test and try the oils through free offers and samples.

One of first and foremost things that vendors and purchasers consider while buying scented or essential oils, apart from the fragrance is the packages. Attractive packages present substandard quality oils, which the products could sell more than the higher quality oils. Moreover pricing is an essential process of the decision making. Vendors typically search in the middle, lower-middle, and related sections, targeting society's favorites. The price and package then is a demand that must meet modest requirements.

The oils do not have to be dressed in fancy package, yet the oils must present some attraction. The demand for aromatherapy in society is based on price driven and high volumes of oils sold. Thus vendors must meet the demand of supplies sold and society's likings.

Denise Williams
How do vendors determine the best way to market aromatherapy?

The average method vendors consider for marketing aromatherapy products is to advertise where customers frequent. Local supermarkets, all-needs stores, flyers, pharmacies, etc are just a few areas that customers visit often. Vendors may also consider targeting the upper middle sections, which they will promote the products, airing them on television or in global and local newspapers.

Vendors will also offer free samples in high-fashioned stores. Since the stores tend to sell fashion accessories for the upper middle class people, vendors assume that the fragrance will sell. The elite sections are another area where vendors promote aromatherapy oils. Choosing aromatherapy essential and scented oils can be problematic, if you do not understand what orals can do for you.

How do I find aromatherapy oils?

Online you can select from favorite oils. Designed scents are available to drown out all your daily stress. Aromatherapy oils assist in helping you relax. As well, aromatherapy oils are available to put you in a romantic mood.

Scented oils can also be utilized to decorate your home, which will warm the environment. The mists of the oils will fill the area with fresh and natural odors.

About Aromatherapy Scented and Essential Oils

Aromatherapy scented and essential oils create a peaceful and loving atmosphere. The oils set the mood while reducing stress from today's over consumed society. When you work all day you will enjoy a moment of relaxation with aromatherapy. Aromatherapy scented oils and essential oils can produce outstanding feelings, whilst enhancing your mood. The scented oils unsurprisingly trigger the physical and tender feelings that a person will express. The aromas set the mood.

How do I choose oils that will set a romantic mood for my partner?

Your partner will enjoy a romantic evening with aromatherapies Jasmine scents. Aromatherapies Jasmine is the emperor of essential oils. Jasmines scented aroma expresses a loving bond, which your mate will likely enjoy. Jasmine is not reserved, and the oil is irresistible. The scent will definitely allure your mate into your arms.

Aromatherapy oils aroma spreads all about your home. The scented oil will appeal to your mate's mood. As well, the oils will ignite the memory, and wet the appetite, as well as the body and mind. Jasmine, as well as other aromatherapy oils are like no other scented or essential oils on the market. The scented and essential oils come in a variety of fragrances and scents. Jasmine, Lilac, Cedar, Myrrh, Tuberose, Rosemary, floral scents, carrier, Absinthe, AJOWAN, African Bluegrass, ANETHI, etc, are just to name a few aromatherapy oils available to you. Angelica Root, Bay, Basil, Anise Star, Australian Balm/Mint Bush, ASAFOETIDA, etc, are other types of aromatherapy oils available on the market.

How do I choose aromatherapy oils that make me want to feel cheery although I am happy?

If you are feeling in good spirits you can stay in the mood by considering the warmth of fig, orange and cinnamon oils. The scented oils will supply you with the natural feelings or moods merely by smelling the oils aroma. The oils can also be utilized as air fresheners. Oils which include chemicals can affect the nasal. As well the chemical based oils can affect regions of the body. Thus,

Denise Williams
non-chemical based oils can make your senses express your moods organically.

Aromatherapy oils produce a sweet aroma, which circulates in the air. However, the oils will not influence your skin in a negative light. In addition, you will not have to invest in products sold in general stockpiles, which refreshes the air artificially. Now you can refresh your home naturally with aromatherapy oils.

How do I choose healing aromatherapy oils?

The aromatherapy botanical oils are ideal for healing. The oils are steam distilled and derive from tree barks. Cinnamon oils are one of aromatherapies scented and essential oils that is made of cinnamon tree barks. The oils come from evergreen native lands, such as Vietnam and China.

CHAPTER 6- A LOOK AT AROMATHERAPY OILS & BLENDS

Costus root's Latin name is Sassuriea Costus. The oils were extracted from plant roots and processed via steam. The India based oils grow black flowers, which the dried plant roots are separated, softened, and soaked in warm water. The plants are then made into Costus root through the steam distillation process.

The oils are brown or yellow, and the common use is to work as an antiseptic, antiviral, febrifuge, antispasmodic, bactericidal, and so on. The oils are claimed to heal those dealing with hypertension, stomach acids, and so on. In addition, Costus root oils is used to make perfumes and cosmetics. Costus roots are also an ingredient in Soda pops and alcohol, as well as in specific foods. The soft aromas blend with Ylang oils, floral scents, patchouli, Oriental oils, and so on. Costus Root however is a dermal irritant, which is not recommended as an aromatherapy.

Coriander essential oils also named Corriandrum Sativum was extracted via the steam distillation process from plant seeds. The Russia based oil produces aroma from its plant. The plants are from the native lands of Asia and throughout Mediterranean areas, and are grown for the purpose of its aromatic leaves. The aroma is also used in cooking. The oils are also called Chinese parsley. Coriander oils are clear or pale yellow and are commonly used as an aphrodisiac, analgesic, deodorant, antispasmodic, and so on.

The oils relieve mental fatigue, rheumatism, nervous disorders, tension, migraines, arthritis, colds, flu, muscle spasms, and so on. The medium strength aromas blend with cinnamon, orange, pink or white oils, ginger, lemon, and so on. The people throughout the lands of Egypt used Coriander more so as an aphrodisiac. India used the oils as a flavoring for foods, while the Greeks and Romans used the oils to flavor their wine.

Copaiba Balsam is another of the essential oils known as Copaifera Officinalis. The oils were steam distilled extracted from crude resin plants. Copaiba Balsam begun in Brazil, yet the oils are now spread throughout the country. The pale yellow oils are commonly used to balance, soothe and uplift the mind and body. Blended aromatherapy oils used with Copaiba Balsam is said to extend life. The medium strength oils blend with spicy oils, floral oils, etc. The oil also has an aphrodisiac agent, which works well with Jasmine, sandalwood, rose, frankincense, vanilla, Ylang oils, and so on. The oils are also used in colognes, soap, perfumes, detergents, and so on.

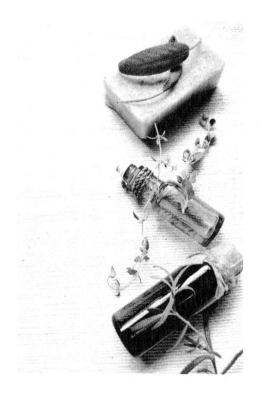

Clove Bud oils named Syzgium Aromaticum as well, came from India. The oils were extracted via steam distillation methods from plant buds. The aromatic spices present a strong aromatic scent, which were distilled from the dried flower buds of the tropical clove trees and used as a flavoring for sweet and spicy foods. The evergreen trees come from the family of myrtle, and from native Moluccas. In addition, the buds are grown in various tropical regions. The light golden yellow oils are commonly used as a treatment for mild aches and pains, such as tooth aches, etc. The oils will help fight colds and flu as well. The scents come in both medium and strong and blend with spicy oils, peppermint, grapefruit, Citronella, Rosemary, rose, orange oils, and lemon oils.

Clementine is an essential oil sometimes known as Citrus Nobilis. The oils were extracted from crude plant peels and through a cold press procedure. The plant originated in Italy. The pale yellow oils are commonly used to revitalize the soul, whilst balancing sleep. Insomniacs could benefit from using this oil. The medium strength oil blends with floral and citrus family scents.

Aromatherapy Blends

Botanic oils include Salvia Sclarea, otherwise known as Clary Sage. The oil was extracted via a steam distillation process, extracted from plant flowers and leaves. The Bulgaria based plants are herbs with hairy-like leaves, and are large in form. The oils extracted from the plants are light golden yellow. The oil is commonly used as an aromatherapy, including used as an antidepressant, sedative, antispasmodic, tonic, deodorant, hypertension healer, and so on. The oil has also been known to assist in relieving asthma symptoms and spasms. The medium or strong scented oil blends with a variety of essential oils, including German, bergamot, Roman, chamomile, Cedarwood, Neroli, jasmine, rosewood, lavender, orange, geranium, sandalwood, Ylang oils, and so on.

Citronella Java oils also called Cymbopogon Winterianus comes from the gum plants and is steam distilled, extracted from the plants. The beginning of citronella arrives at Sri Lanka. The lemon aromatic grass is an Asian tropical bluish green, lemon aromatic leave, and contains aromatic oils. The oils are used in perfumes, and are used as an insect repellent. The oils are yellowish brown, and are used as an aromatherapy. The oils include antiseptics, insecticide, deodorant, tonics, and parasitic. Used with Cedarwood flavors the oil can work well as an insect repellent. The oils are also used to make candles, soaps, etc. You can use the oils to fight flu and cols, as well as oily hair/skin and perspiration. The medium scents blend with in variety of oils, including pine, bergamot, lavender, bitter orange, orange, Cedarwood, lemon, and Geranium oils. Still, it is a, predominate insect repellent.

Another of the botanic oils available is the Citral essentials. The oil was extracted via the steam distill process, which came from stems and roots from plants. China is the beginning, yet China is far from the end of this oils roots. The oils are light yellow and commonly used as an antiseptic, invigorator, antidepressant, and works to heal the nerves, and soothe pain and aches. The oil produces a strong lemon scent, as well as an herbaceous scent. The oils will treat athletic foot odors and itching, acne, scabies, oily skin, and will help to reduce stress.

The botanic aromatherapy Chilly Seed oils were distilled from steam and plant seeds. The Mexico based oils also comes from plants in Southern America and Central America. The rich, reddish orange oils are commonly used in aromatherapy, since it has an analgesic agent, anti-inflammatory agent, and an aid to the digestive system. The strong scents do not blend with other oils.

When you are searching for aromatherapy oils it is best to shop online. Shopping online gives you advantages, including live

Essential Oils Bible

support. In other words, you can find Live Chat Support online to help you find oils that may not be listed in the series of articles. I thought I would throw this in to give you a briefing on how shopping online can bring you a variety of benefits.

Continuing Chenopodium essential oils were extracted from plant fruit and leaves and distilled through the use of steam. The Russia based oils are commonly used in a variety of problems. The oils will work to remove roundworms, Ascaride, as well as treat diuretics. The strong scent does not blend with other oils. The oils are sometime called the American Wormseed Oils.

Choulmogra is another of the essential oils utilized in treating rheumatism, skin disease, eczema, scrofula, bruising, sores, sprains, leprosy, and so on. The oil derived from India but is currently utilized all over the world.

CHAPTER 7- BOTANIC EXTRACTS FOR AROMATHERAPY

Botanic extracts in aromatherapy product line are 100% natural. The powered extracts are ideal for using as toiletry, and to treat hair and skin. The extracts compose biology cells, which serve as a purpose to structure. The extracts compose organic salts, fats, amino acids, minerals and oils. The extracts include cucumber, barley grass, green tea extracts, chamomile, lotus leaf, St. John, Ginseng, and so on. Additional blends include the Reishi Mushroom, White Willow, Gentian Root, Bilberry, Guarana seed, and so on.

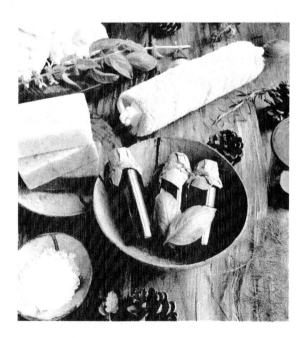

Online you will find a variety of extracts, essential oils, scented oils, fragrances, and more along the aromatherapy product line. Aromatherapy has long line of essential oils, yet all the oils listed are not aromatherapy solutions.

Some of the oils include absinthe, ajowan, African bluegrass, anethi, Angelica root, anise star, armoise mugwort, arborvitae wild, asafoetida, basil, Australian balm mint brush, bay, bergamot, bay, Betal leaf, Blood orange, black currant seed, Cajeput, Cade, and so on. The oils work in a variety of ways to soothe and heal the body and mind.

Blood orange is an essential oil, which comes from the citrus family. The oil was extracted through a cold press method. The oils come from crude plant fruit peels and it originated in Italy. The deep orange oils are commonly used as aromatherapy relieving a variety of illnesses. The oils include an antispasmodic, antidepressant, deodorant, aphrodisiac, cordial, nervous stimulants, digestive, cardiac, and circulatory stimulants, as well as carminative aids. The medium scent oils blend with myrrh, nutmeg, lemon, lavender, clove, clary sage, cinnamon, etc. Blood orange is sometimes called Maltese Orange. Spanish natives continue to call the oils Naranja.

Ajowan another of aromatherapy's essential oils, stems from herbs and are extracted from a steam distill method. The starting point of ajowan oils come from India. Ajowan oils are pale yellow, brown. Ajowan oils are basic for motivating the body and mind. As well ajowan is exploited as an antispasmodic remedy. AS add-on ajowan oil have microscopic organisms, in addition to properties, which assist in fighting bellyaches, cramps, heartburn, or related colic symptoms. Ajowan has a strong scent what blends with sage, parsley and the aromatic plants known as thymes.

Chamomile Roman oils derived from Hungary, and are processed through a steam distillation, which the oils are extracted from flower head plants. The yellow oils are commonly used as an ingredient in herbal medicines. The oils are useful in treating insomnia, aches and pains, joint and muscle discomforts, PMS, etc.

The strong aroma scents aid as relaxant, sedative, and disinfect. The oil blends with lavender, frankincense, geranium, rosewood, rose, clary sage, marjoram, Ylang oils, Cedarwood, and so on.

Australian balms oils assist in helping relieve headaches, colds, bellyaches, including colic symptoms, and so on. The oil's Latin name is Prostandthera Melissifolia. Like many other of aromatherapy's oils the plants were extracted through a steam process. The oil includes an antibacterial solution. The oils also have anti-fungal agents.

Bay essential oils come from the leaves of particular plants and are steamed distilled. The plants derive from West India. The plants are also grown in Guiana and Venezuela. The golden yellow oils produced from the Bay plants aid as an antiseptic, astringent, antibiotic, analgesic, aperitif, anti-neuralgic, and so on. You can use oil to rest rheumatism symptoms, neuralgia, circulation discomforts, flu, colds, muscle pain, skin infections, dental infections, and diarrhea. The strong oils blend with juniper, cedar wood, ginger, Ylang oils, geranium, Rosemary, rose, orange scents, lemon, eucalyptus, thyme, coriander, etc. The sweet smelling aromas are said to symbolize peace, wisdom, and security. Bay oils are also used to make rum liquors. Using aromatherapy in healing is becoming a huge action.

CHAPTER 8- TOP CHOICE AROMATHERAPY OILS

Aromatherapy expressions include the top choice oils. The oils lemon, bergamot, lavender, orange sweet, tea tree, lemongrass, eucalyptus, lavender French, rosemary French, and peppermint Japanese are the top oils sold at various companies.

What Do Lemon Oils Do?

Lemon scents are botanical oils, which is from the citrus family. The oils are cold pressed (Expressions) and extracted from peels of fruits. The plants derived from Italy; however, California, Europe, Florida, and India cultivate the plants as well. The light color oils are used to cleanse, and is famous for its antiseptic base. The oil cools and refreshes the body and mind, as well and enhances concentration. The fresh lemon scents also incorporate anti-bacterial agents, which work to heal the hair and skin. During the Middle Ages European natives frequently used lemon oils. In addition, Romans and the Greeks used lemon oils as aromatherapy.

What about Lavender Oils?

Lavender oils work to clarify, balance, regulate, and soothe the body and mind. Lavender oils include Population, Australian, Mont Blanc, Barreme, French, Bulgarian, Croatian, and 40/42.

The 40/42 oils stems from Latin Lavandula Officinalis, which the flower heads are steamed condensed in 40 to 42% Ester. The origin of Lavender 40/42 is France. The plants grow violet, mauve, purple, blue lilacs. The plants produce pale yellow, or tinted green oils. Lavender 40/42 is commonly used as a therapeutic treatment. Included in lavender is analgesic, anti-microbial, anti-convulsant, antidepressant, antiseptic, antitoxic, etc. The oils are used to treat hypertension, diuretic, and so on. Lavender is used in perfumes, soaps, cosmetics, candles, etc. Lavender 40/42 has a strong scent, which blends with the majority of aromatherapy oils. Floral, clove, citrus, pine, cedar wood, patchouli, labdanum, clary sage, Vetiver, etc are to name a few.

Bergamot essential oils is one the top sellers. The oil helps to relieve stress related symptoms, such as fear, nervousness, hysteria, anxiety, and fatigue. In addition, the oils will assist in treating bronchitis, migraines, congested skin, arthritis, etc. The strong scented oils include Bergaptene Free, in which the oils are referred as Bergamot Citrus. The oils are extracted via the cold press method, or expressions. The fruit peels make up bergamot oils, which derive from Italy.

The oils are Asia based spiny citrus trees, which grow tart shaped pears. The Latina name is Citrus Bergamia. Aromatherapy bergamot oils are yellow, green. The fruits rinds were utilized to create the bergamot oils, which include perfumes. Akin to bergamot are the Mediterranean mint plants. Bergamot is said to heal or relieve depression, fear, hysteria, anorexia, anxiety, eczema, various infections, psoriasis, and so on. Bergaptene also works as a healer. The aromas produce medium scents, which blend with Rosemary, Mandarin, Cypress oils, Frankincense, Clary Sage, Nutmeg, and so on. Sandalwood, orange, Ylang oils, Jasmine oils, etc all work with Bergamia blends.

Tea Tree oils come from Australia, and are steamed distilled from plant leaves. The Tea Tree Australian makes tea. As well the trees are partner to New Zealand trees and shrubs. The leaves were formally utilized to make tea, however a wide production of oils are made from the trees today, as well cosmetics, lotions, etc are made from the Tea Trees, which is used as an antiseptic. Tea Tree is commonly used as essential oils, which has a powerful immunity stimulator. Tea Tree fights infectious organisms, such as fungi, bacteria, and various viruses. Tea Tree is used as massage oil, which helps to reduce pre-operation shock. The oils in massage therapy serve as a therapy. AS well, the Tea Tree oils fight colds, sinus interruptions, measles, viral infections, etc. You can use tea tree oils to treat your hair and skin as well. Continue reading to learn more about foreign aromatherapy oils.

CHAPTER 9- THE LINK BETWEEN AROMATHERAPY AND MASSAGE THERAPY

Aromatherapy started as a combination of massage and essential oils, however the essential oils broke away from massage therapy and now the oils are acting as standalones to heal the body and mind? About 6000 years ago, the Egyptian doctors recommended aromatherapy through massage. The practices helped to relieve aches, pains, and reduce stress. Later, massage and aromatherapy was also recommended as the better solution to enforce a healthier mind and body. The question then, is how can essential oils standalone to fight diseases and heal the body and mind?

Essential oils are any members of the volatile oils, which give characteristic to plants, such as oils which are used as flavorings and perfumes. Essential oils differ from fixed oils, since the fixed oils are non-fatty and non-volatile.

Then, how can I tell if essential oils will work as stand alones compared to massage?

We can consider massage therapy vs. aromatherapy essential oils to see if the oils are capable of standing alone to heal the body and mind. First, I want to say that this is a good question because most people may find it hard to believe that essential oils could stand alone to heal the body and mind.

Massage

Massage therapy incorporates reflexology and manipulation while pressing down and rubbing the body. The process is a kneading action, which the masseuse will focus on pressure points. That is, a good masseuse will focus on pressure points. If you hit the right pressure points you can release tension in the stomach area, around the lower back, shoulders, etc. If you combine essential oils you will set an atmosphere, which will promote relaxation. The natural scents set the mood.

Stand-Alone Essential Oils

Essential oils work in as stand-alones; we see can set the mood by using natural aromatic scents that circulate the atmosphere. Essential oils are naturally extracted and are made from plants or its materials, which the plants fundamental properties are preserved, e.g. flavors and fragrance. Since the plants and its materials come from natural sources why would it not help the body and mind to relax? Well, let's see. What do aromatherapy essential oils claim to do?

Fir needle is one of the essential oils available. The oils come from an evergreen tree, which grows leaves shaped like needles. The leaves erect from a female cone. The Siberian tree itself resembles fir. Now, according to marketers this oil can assist in healing bronchitis symptoms, colds, flu, coughing, sinusitis, arthritis, rheumatism, and muscle aches and pains. According to reports the oils natural ingredients were preserved, such as antiseptics. Antiseptics we know are antibacterial properties, which deliver uncontaminated, clean, and pure solutions. Now imagine breathing antiseptics from aromatherapy scents? If the source is uncontaminated, pure, and clean why would, it not gives some kind of effect, such as good results? This is especially true if you are inhaling the antiseptic from the air.

Frankincense is another of aromatherapy's essential oils. The oil derives from aromatic resin. The gum and/or resin are commonly burned as incense. AS well, it is distilled, preserved and added to

Denise Williams

perfume. In fact, many religious ceremonies use this incense at their gatherings. This particular scent is an aromatherapy solution, which its properties include antiseptics. Again, we can breathe this preserved property in the air, which could help resolve diuretic, astringent, remove tonic, etc. In fact, it could even act as a sedative, since if your symptoms are relieved, why would, you not relax.

CONCLUSION

Aromatherapy incorporates essential oils to deliver a therapeutic solution. The solutions have been used throughout the years by Egyptians, Russians, Spain, Brazil, Europe, Canadians, French, Germany, India, etc. Any remedy I feel coming from overseas has sometime to offer, since these people have remedies available that has proven to work, yet the US Government and FDA will not allow the remedies into the US. There has to be a reason, and that reason is money.

Aromatherapy remedies are claimed to relieve symptoms coming from a variety of diseases. The essential oils are claimed to relieve stress, anxiety, nervous tension, and related symptoms. The oils include the scented and essential oils. Online you can find a variety of the oils, including Basil, cedar wood, celery seed, carrot seed, African Bluegrass oils, bergamot, clove bud and leaf oils, and so on. The oils each have its purpose for healing the body and mind. Before using the oils be, sure to read all available instructions before using. In conclusion, learn about the products you are considering before purchasing to make sure you are getting the natural oils.

ABOUT THE AUTHOR

Denise Williams has always had a love for all things natural. She grew up in a home where her parents practiced the sustainable lifestyle as such they grew most of their own foods and her mother used herbs to cure common ailments.

She carried this philosophy into her own lifestyle and as a result of this she embraced the thought of using essential oils for the host of benefits that come with it.

CPSIA information can be obtained
at www.ICGtesting.com
Printed in the USA
LVOW03s2300050417
529690LV00015B/516/P